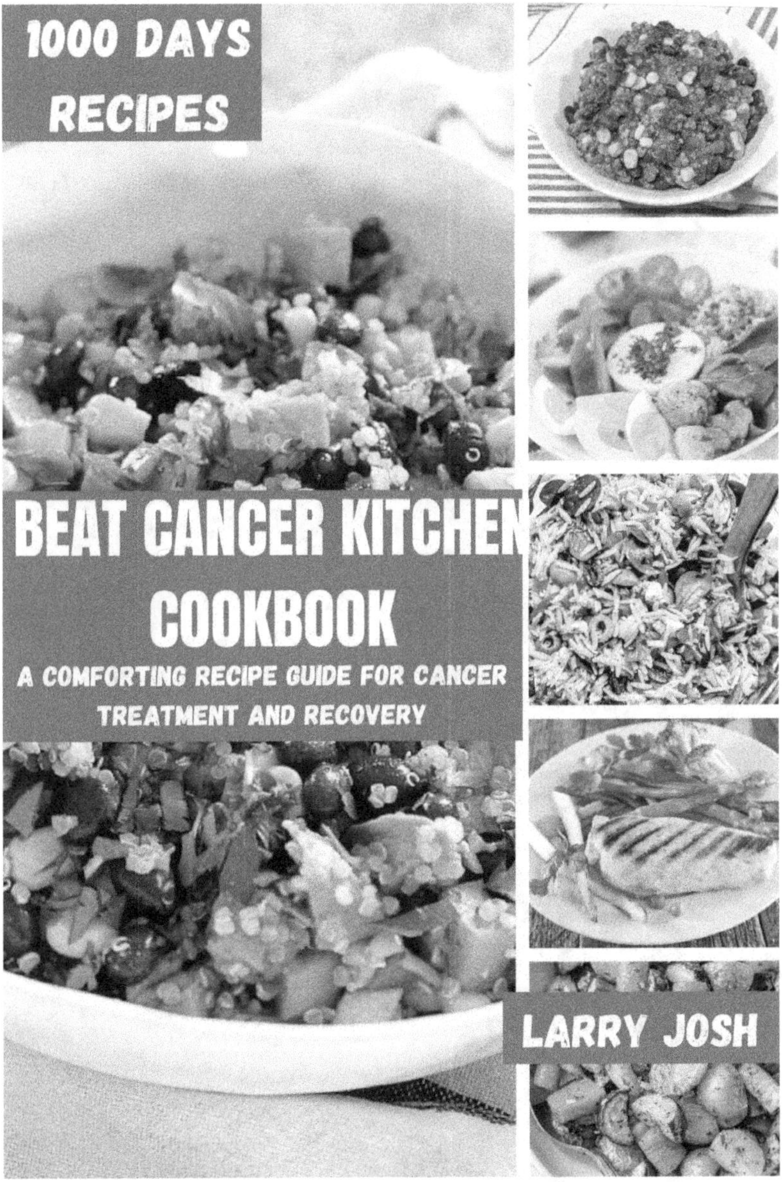

1000 DAYS RECIPES

BEAT CANCER KITCHEN COOKBOOK

A COMFORTING RECIPE GUIDE FOR CANCER TREATMENT AND RECOVERY

LARRY JOSH

Beat Cancer Kitchen Cookbook

By Larry Josh

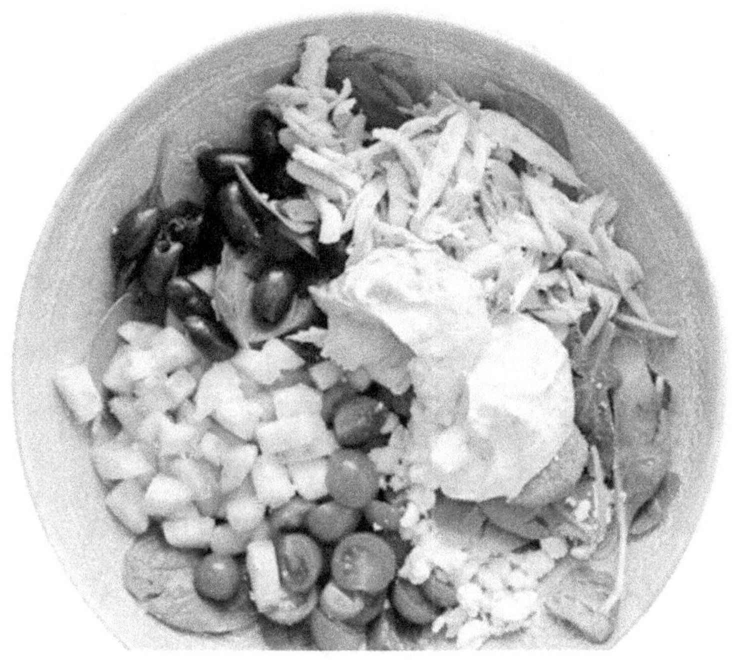

A Comforting Recipe Guide for Cancer Treatment and Recovery

Copyright 2024/Larry Josh. All rights reserved.

All Rights Reserved Under International Copyright Law.

No Part of this cookbook may be reproduced or transmitted in any form or by any means, electronic or mechanical including photocopying, recording, or by any information storage and retrieval system without permission in writing from the publisher.

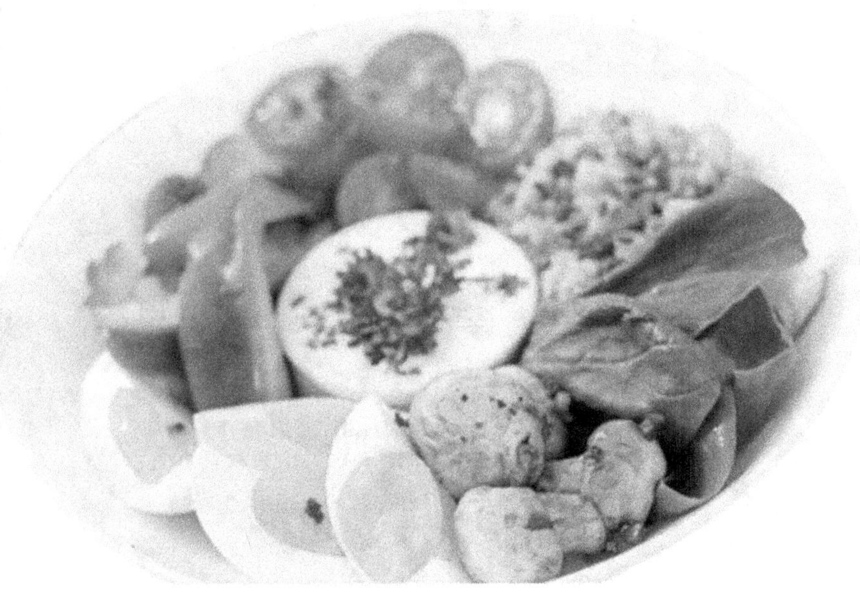

As the author of this amazing recipe cookbook, I will love to let you know that your good health is my priority. Please take your time to read through this book step by step. May the LORD bless us and keep us as you do so.
AMEN

NOW LET'S COOK

Table Of Contents

Chapter 1. Introduction

Understanding Cancer

Cancer, a formidable adversary, disrupts lives and introduces unexpected challenges. It's a complex puzzle that reshapes not only our physical health but also our daily experiences.

Impact on Body Systems

This insidious force alters the delicate balance within the body's systems. From the intricate battles within our cells to the broader effects on immunity and organ function, cancer weaves its impact through every aspect of our being.

Purpose of the Cookbook

In response to this formidable foe, we present the "Beat Cancer Kitchen Cookbook." It's more than a compilation of recipes; it's a caring guide crafted to provide comfort, nourishment, and unwavering support throughout the demanding journey of cancer treatment and recovery.

Impact of Nutrition on Cancer Treatment

Within these pages lies a recognition of the transformative power of nutrition. This cookbook explores how a thoughtful and well-balanced diet can significantly influence the body's ability to navigate the complexities of cancer treatment. It goes beyond ingredients; it's a step towards building resilience, embracing healing, and offering solace to both body and soul.

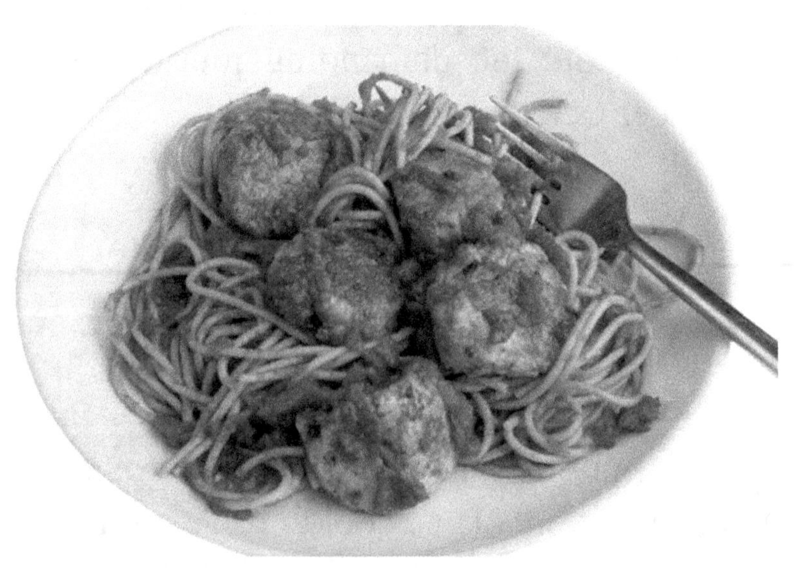

Chapter 2.
Understanding Cancer and Nutrition

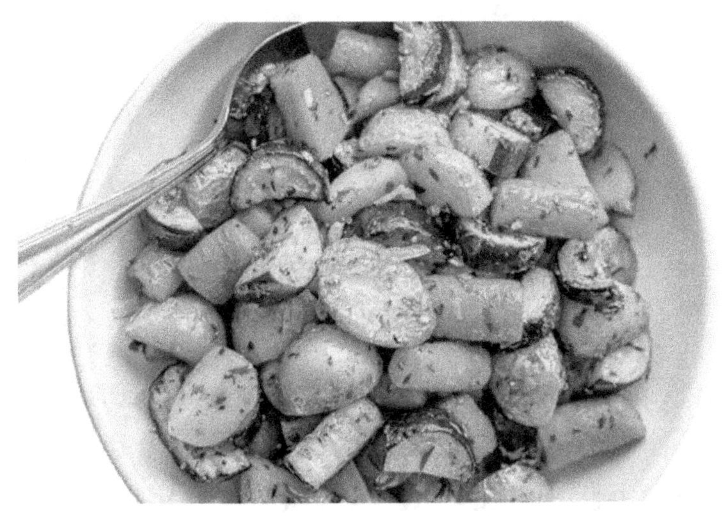

In this chapter, we're delving into the intricate interplay between what we eat and the formidable force that is cancer. Think of it as unraveling a puzzle—one where the choices on our plate can influence the complex pathways of cancer development and progression. This knowledge is not just about understanding; it's about empowering you to make informed dietary decisions as you navigate the challenging terrain of cancer.

The Connection Between Cancer and Diet

At the heart of our exploration is the fundamental connection between our dietary habits and the intricate dance of cancer within our bodies. We're starting with the basics—how cells grow, divide, and sometimes go rogue. From there, we're diving into the vibrant world of fruits and vegetables, exploring how the antioxidants in them might just be the superheroes disrupting cancer's plans. This section aims to shed light on how the food we choose can influence the battleground within our bodies, potentially tipping the scales in our favor.

Importance of a Well-Balanced Diet During Treatment

As we transition into the realm of cancer treatment, the significance of a well-balanced diet becomes even more pronounced. Undergoing treatments like chemotherapy and radiation places an immense strain on the body. Now, more than ever, the role of a well-balanced diet transforms into a vital support system. It's about aiding recovery, bolstering the immune system, and providing the essential strength needed to confront and overcome the disease. This is not just about filling our stomachs; it's about strategically nourishing our bodies for resilience and healing in the face of cancer's challenges.

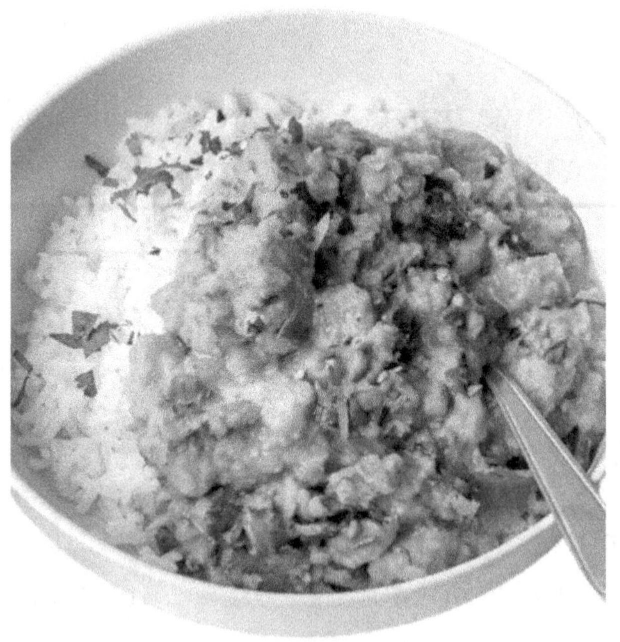

Chapter 3. Building a Cancer Beat Kitchen

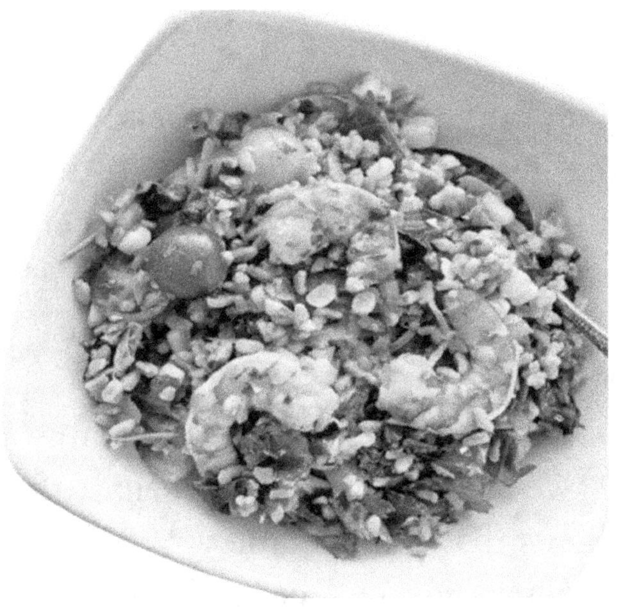

In the heart of the culinary journey towards beating cancer lies the essential foundation of building a well-equipped kitchen. This chapter is not just about recipes; it's about creating a space that empowers you, ensuring that every meal becomes a step towards resilience and healing.

Essential Ingredients and Pantry Staples

Picture your kitchen as a canvas, and the ingredients within it as the vibrant palette. To build a Beat Cancer Kitchen, we'll explore the essential elements—foods that are not just flavorful but also packed with nutrients. From fresh produce to wholesome grains, we'll delve into the arsenal of ingredients that can become your allies in the fight against cancer. Additionally, we'll stock up your pantry with staples that form the backbone of nutritious meals, making it easier for you to craft nourishing dishes with minimal hassle.

Kitchen Tools for Easy Preparation:

Now that we've filled our kitchen with the right ingredients, let's equip it with the tools that make preparation a breeze. The goal here is simplicity. We'll explore kitchen gadgets and utensils that streamline the cooking process, making it accessible even during moments of fatigue. From sharp knives that cut through effortlessly to easy-to-use appliances that save time, we're creating a kitchen space that works with you, not against you.

As we embark on this chapter, envision your kitchen as a sanctuary—a place where healing ingredients and practical tools come together to create not just meals but moments of strength and nourishment. Welcome to the Beat Cancer Kitchen, where every element is carefully chosen to support you on your journey towards health and well-being.

Chapter 4. Mindful Cooking and Eating

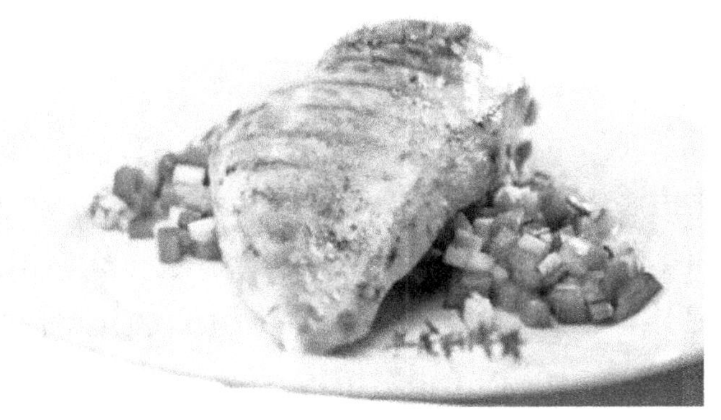

In the rhythmic dance of preparing and consuming food, lies a powerful ally in the journey towards beating cancer. This chapter is an exploration of mindfulness—an intentional approach to cooking and eating that transcends the simple act of nourishing the body. It's about being present, savoring each moment, and finding a profound connection between the food on your plate and your well-being.

Benefits of Mindful Eating

Mindful eating is not just about what's on your plate; it's about how you approach every bite. In this section, we'll uncover the transformative benefits of being fully present during meals. From enhancing digestion to fostering a healthier relationship with food, mindful eating becomes a tool for both physical and emotional well-being. We'll explore how this intentional practice can bring a sense of calm to your dining experience, encouraging a deeper connection with the nourishment your body receives.

Incorporating Mindfulness into Cooking

Cooking is not merely a chore but an art—a mindful practice that can be therapeutic and uplifting. In this part, we'll delve into the art of incorporating mindfulness into your culinary endeavors. From the rhythmic chopping of vegetables to the gentle simmering of a comforting broth, we'll explore how being fully present during the cooking process can elevate the nourishment of both body and soul. It's not just about the end result; it's about finding joy and tranquility in the act of creating a meal.

As we enter the realm of mindful cooking and eating, envision it as a journey—one where each mindful bite and every intentional stir of the spoon becomes a step towards healing and embracing the fullness of the present moment. Welcome to a chapter where your kitchen becomes a haven for mindfulness, and each meal becomes a celebration of life and well-being.

Chapter 5. Healing Broths and Comforting Soups

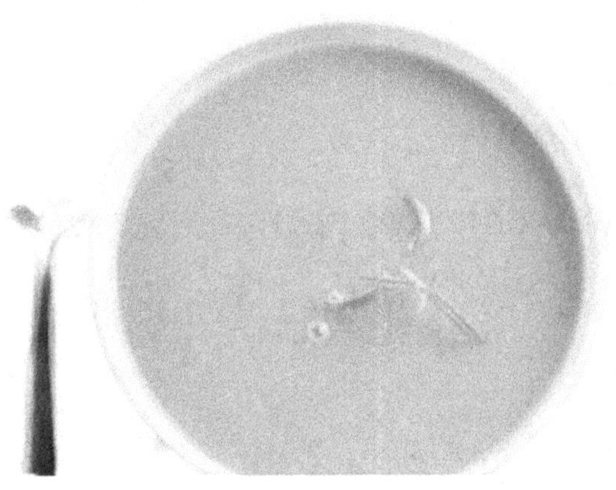

In the world of culinary comfort, few dishes rival the soothing embrace of healing broths and comforting soups. This chapter is a journey into warmth and nourishment, exploring the therapeutic qualities of broths and the heartening nature of a well-crafted soup. It's not just about flavors; it's about the healing power that steams from a comforting bowl.

Soup 1: Nourishing Chicken and Vegetable Broth

Ingredients:

1 whole chicken, preferably organic

Assorted vegetables (carrots, celery, onion)

Fresh ginger, peeled and sliced

Garlic cloves, crushed

Bay leaves and a handful of fresh herbs (rosemary, thyme)

Salt and pepper to taste

Preparation:

Place the chicken in a large pot and cover with water.

Add chopped vegetables, ginger, garlic, bay leaves, and herbs.

Bring to a boil, then reduce heat and simmer for at least 2 hours.

Season with salt and pepper. Strain the broth and discard solids.

Enjoy the soothing warmth of this nourishing chicken and vegetable broth.

Soup 2: Lentil and Spinach Comfort Soup

Ingredients:

1 cup dried green or brown lentils

Onion, finely chopped

Carrots, diced

Celery, sliced

Fresh spinach leaves, roughly chopped

Garlic cloves, minced

Vegetable broth

Cumin, coriander, and turmeric for seasoning

Olive oil for sautéing

Preparation:

Sauté onions, carrots, celery, and garlic in olive oil until softened.

Add lentils, vegetable broth, and spices. Bring to a boil.

Reduce heat and simmer until lentils are tender.

Stir in fresh spinach and cook until wilted.

Ladle into bowls and relish the wholesome goodness of this lentil and spinach comfort soup.

Soup 3: Creamy Butternut Squash Elixir

Ingredients:

Butternut squash, peeled and diced

Onion, chopped

Carrots, chopped

Vegetable broth

Coconut milk

Fresh thyme leaves

Nutmeg, salt, and pepper to taste

Preparation:

Sauté onions, carrots, and butternut squash until softened.

Add vegetable broth, thyme, and bring to a simmer until vegetables are tender.

Blend until smooth, then stir in coconut milk.

Season with nutmeg, salt, and pepper.

Savor the velvety richness of this creamy butternut squash elixir.

These soul-warming soups are crafted not just for taste but for the comfort and nourishment they bring. Each spoonful is a step towards healing and a reminder that, in a bowl of soup, lies a universe of wellness.

Chapter 6. Gentle and Nutrient Dense Dishes

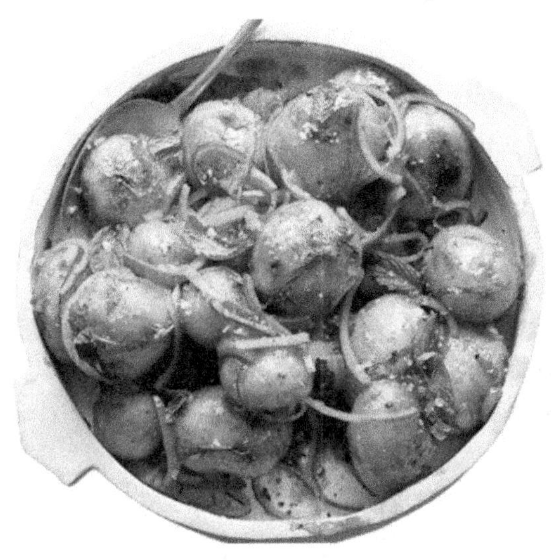

As we navigate the culinary landscape tailored for those seeking comfort and nourishment during challenging times, we enter the realm of "Gentle and Nutrient-Dense Dishes." This chapter is a thoughtful collection of recipes designed to be not only palatable but also easily digestible, offering a wealth of essential nutrients without compromising on flavor or comfort.

Soup 1: Quinoa and Vegetable Delight

Ingredients

Quinoa, rinsed

Mixed vegetables (zucchini, bell peppers, carrots), diced

Onion, finely chopped

Garlic cloves, minced

Low-sodium vegetable broth

Fresh parsley, chopped

Lemon juice, for a refreshing twist

Olive oil for sautéing

Preparation

Sauté onions, garlic, and mixed vegetables in olive oil until softened.

Add quinoa and vegetable broth, bringing it to a boil.

Reduce heat and simmer until quinoa is cooked.

Stir in fresh parsley and a splash of lemon juice.

Serve this delightful quinoa and vegetable soup as a nutrient-packed meal.

Soup 2: Silken Miso Tofu Bowl

Ingredients:

Silken tofu, cubed

Wakame seaweed, soaked and chopped

Scallions, thinly sliced

Low-sodium vegetable broth

White miso paste

Mirin for sweetness (optional)

Sesame oil for flavor

Soy sauce, to taste

Preparation:

In a pot, combine vegetable broth, miso paste, and mirin (if using).

Bring to a gentle simmer, then add tofu, wakame, and scallions.

Cook until the tofu is heated through.

Season with soy sauce and a drizzle of sesame oil.

Enjoy the delicate balance of flavors in this silken miso tofu bowl.

Soup 3: Easy Lentil and Sweet Potato Stew

Ingredients:

Red lentils, rinsed

Sweet potatoes, peeled and diced

Onion, diced

Garlic cloves, minced

Low-sodium vegetable broth

Ground cumin and coriander

Smoked paprika for depth

Fresh cilantro, chopped, for garnish

Preparation:

Sauté onions and garlic until softened.

Add sweet potatoes, lentils, vegetable broth, and spices.

Bring to a boil, then simmer until lentils and sweet potatoes are tender.

Garnish with fresh cilantro before serving.

Dive into the heartiness of this easy lentil and sweet potato stew, brimming with nutrients.

These gentle and nutrient-dense dishes are crafted with care, offering a blend of comforting textures and essential goodness. With each spoonful, experience the embrace of flavors that contribute not only to your palate but also to your overall well-being.

Chapter 7. Hydrating Beverage and Snacks

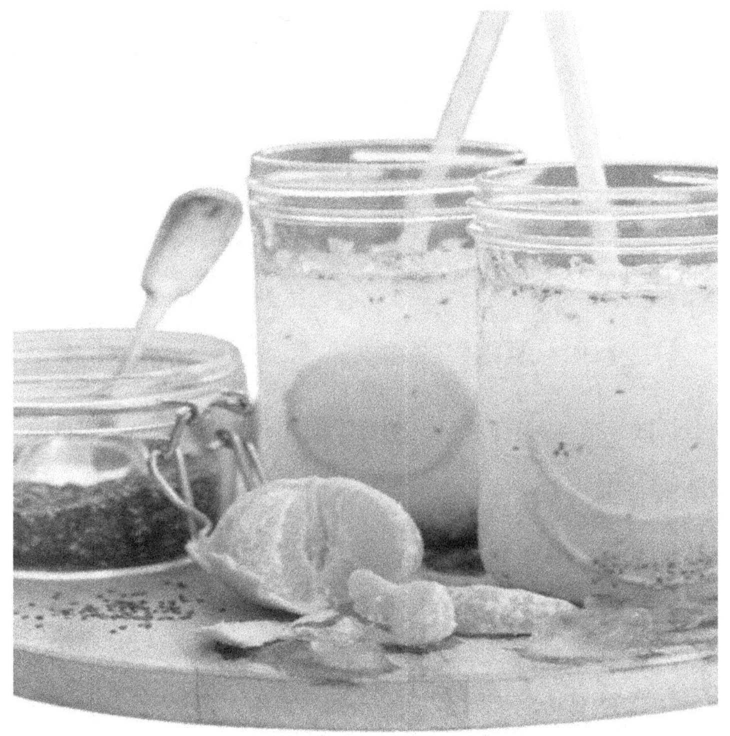

As we venture into Chapter 7, a haven of rejuvenation awaits in "Hydrating Beverages and Snacks." Here, we explore a collection of refreshing elixirs and satisfying bites designed to keep you nourished, hydrated, and uplifted during the challenging journey of cancer treatment and recovery.

Hydrating Beverage 1: Citrus Mint Infusion

Ingredients:

Fresh citrus slices (lemon, lime, orange)

Fresh mint leaves

Cucumber, thinly sliced

Ice cubes

Sparkling water

Preparation:

In a pitcher, combine citrus slices, mint leaves, and cucumber.

Add ice cubes for a refreshing chill.

Pour sparkling water over the mixture.

Stir gently and let it infuse for a few minutes.

Serve this invigorating citrus mint infusion to stay hydrated with a burst of flavor.

Hydrating Beverage 2: Berry Blast Smoothie

Ingredients:

Mixed berries (strawberries, blueberries, raspberries)

Greek yogurt

Almond milk

Chia seeds

Honey for sweetness

Ice cubes

Preparation:

Blend mixed berries, Greek yogurt, and almond milk until smooth.

Add chia seeds and honey to taste.

Throw in a handful of ice cubes and blend again.

Pour this vibrant berry blast smoothie into a glass.

Sip and relish the nutrient-packed goodness of this hydrating delight.

Hydrating Beverage 3: Green Tea and Ginger Elixir

Ingredients:

Green tea bags

Fresh ginger, sliced

Honey for sweetness

Lemon slices

Boiling water

Preparation:

Steep green tea bags and fresh ginger slices in boiling water.

Let it steep for 3-5 minutes.

Add honey to taste and stir.

Garnish with lemon slices.

Enjoy the soothing warmth and antioxidants of this green tea and ginger elixir.

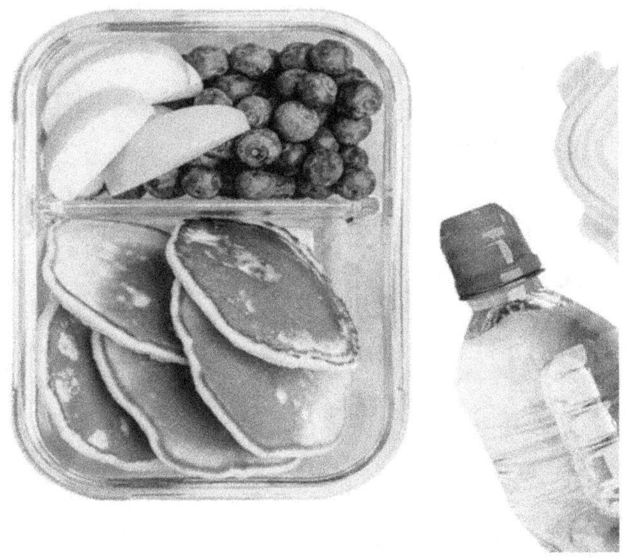

Snack 1: Nutty Energy Bites

Ingredients:

Rolled oats

Nut butter (almond, peanut, or cashew)

Honey or maple syrup for sweetness

Chia seeds

Dark chocolate chips

Shredded coconut for coating

Preparation:

In a bowl, combine rolled oats, nut butter, honey or maple syrup, chia seeds, and chocolate chips.

Mix until well combined.

Form small, bite-sized balls from the mixture.

Roll the balls in shredded coconut for a coating.

Chill in the refrigerator and enjoy these nutty energy bites as a satisfying snack.

Snack 2: Greek Yogurt Parfait

Ingredients:

Greek yogurt

Mixed berries (strawberries, blueberries, raspberries)

Granola

Honey for drizzling

Preparation:

In a glass or bowl, layer Greek yogurt, mixed berries, and granola.

Repeat the layers to your liking.

Drizzle honey on top for sweetness.

Indulge in the delightful textures and flavors of this Greek yogurt parfait.

Snack 3: Hummus and Veggie Sticks

Ingredients:

Hummus (store-bought or homemade)

Carrot and cucumber sticks

Bell pepper strips

Cherry tomatoes

Preparation:

Arrange carrot and cucumber sticks, bell pepper strips, and cherry tomatoes on a plate.

Serve with a bowl of hummus for dipping.

Enjoy the crunch and freshness of this simple yet satisfying hummus and veggie snack.

This chapter unfolds a repertoire of hydrating beverages and snacks, providing not just sustenance but a delightful respite during your cancer journey. Each sip and bite is a moment of refreshment and nourishment, contributing to your overall well-being.

Chapter 8. Family Friends Comfort Foods

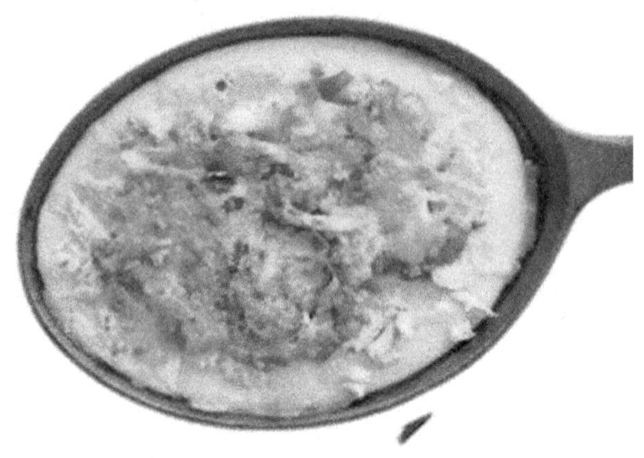

In Chapter 8, we embark on a culinary journey that transcends individual nourishment and extends its embrace to the whole family. "Family-Friendly Comfort Foods" is a collection of hearty, wholesome recipes designed to bring loved ones together around the table, fostering moments of warmth, connection, and nourishment.

Soup 1: Hearty Minestrone for All

Ingredients:

Olive oil

Onion, diced

Carrots, diced

Celery, sliced

Garlic cloves, minced

Cannellini beans, drained and rinsed

Zucchini, diced

Crushed tomatoes

Vegetable broth

Pasta (small shapes)

Fresh basil and Parmesan for garnish

Salt and pepper to taste

Preparation:

In a pot, sauté onions, carrots, celery, and garlic in olive oil until softened.

Add beans, zucchini, crushed tomatoes, and vegetable broth. Bring to a boil.

Stir in pasta and simmer until pasta is cooked.

Season with salt and pepper.

Garnish with fresh basil and Parmesan before serving. Enjoy this hearty minestrone as a family-friendly comfort meal.

Soup 2: Creamy Tomato Basil Bisque

Ingredients:

Butter

Onion, chopped

Carrots, diced

Garlic cloves, minced

Canned whole tomatoes

Vegetable broth

Fresh basil leaves

Heavy cream

Salt and pepper to taste

Croutons for garnish

Preparation:

In a pot, melt butter and sauté onions, carrots, and garlic until softened.

Add canned tomatoes and vegetable broth. Simmer for 20 minutes.

Blend the mixture until smooth. Return to the pot.

Stir in fresh basil and heavy cream. Simmer until heated through.

Season with salt and pepper. Garnish with croutons before serving. Relish the creamy richness of this tomato basil bisque with the family.

Soup 3: Cheesy Broccoli Cheddar Soup

Ingredients:

Butter

Onion, chopped

Carrots, diced

Broccoli florets

Vegetable broth

All-purpose flour

Milk

Sharp cheddar cheese, grated

Nutmeg, salt, and pepper to taste

Preparation:

In a pot, melt butter and sauté onions, carrots, and broccoli until tender.

Sprinkle flour over the veggies and stir to coat.

Pour in vegetable broth and milk. Simmer until thickened.

Add grated cheddar cheese and stir until melted.

Season with nutmeg, salt, and pepper. Serve this cheesy broccoli cheddar soup to warm hearts at the family table.

These family-friendly comfort soups are crafted to unite and nourish. Gather around, share a bowl, and savor the moments of togetherness as these hearty soups bring warmth and comfort to your family table.

Chapter 9.
Customizable Recipes for Individual Needs

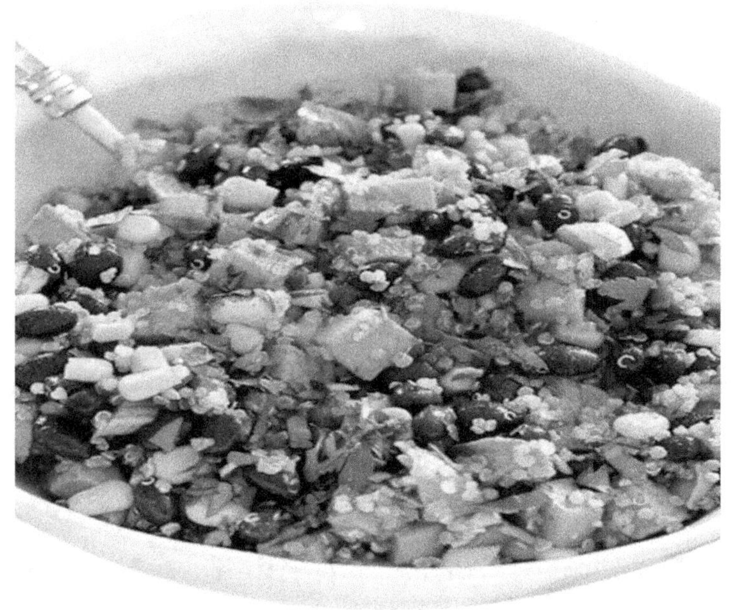

In this chapter, you'll find recipes that embrace the art of customization. From ingredient swaps to portion adjustments, the goal is to provide a framework that empowers you to tailor each dish to your liking. Whether you're exploring plant-based alternatives, adjusting spice levels, or modifying textures, these recipes offer a culinary playground for your creativity.

Customizable Recipe 1: Build-Your-Own Grain Bowl

Ingredients:

Cooked grains (quinoa, rice, farro, or your choice)

Assorted vegetables (bell peppers, cherry tomatoes, cucumbers, avocado)

Protein source (grilled chicken, chickpeas, tofu)

Fresh herbs (cilantro, parsley)

Dressing of choice (lemon vinaigrette, tahini, balsamic glaze)

Preparation:

Arrange a base of cooked grains in a bowl.

Top with a variety of colorful vegetables and your preferred protein.

Sprinkle fresh herbs for added flavor.

Drizzle with your favorite dressing to tie it all together.

Mix and match ingredients to create a personalized grain bowl tailored to your taste.

Customizable Recipe 2: DIY Veggie Wraps

Ingredients:

Whole-grain or gluten-free wraps

Hummus or your preferred spread

Assorted raw and cooked vegetables (lettuce, spinach, shredded carrots, roasted peppers)

Protein choice (grilled chicken, falafel, or beans)

Optional toppings (avocado, feta cheese, olives)

Sauce or dressing of choice

Preparation:

Spread a layer of hummus or your chosen spread on the wrap.

Arrange a variety of fresh and cooked veggies on top.

Add your preferred protein choice.

Sprinkle with optional toppings for extra flair.

Drizzle with your favorite sauce or dressing.

Roll it up and enjoy a customized veggie wrap designed just for you.

Customizable Recipe 3: Adaptable Smoothie Bowl

Ingredients:

Frozen fruit of your choice (berries, mango, banana)

Greek yogurt or plant-based yogurt

Liquid (milk, almond milk, coconut water)

Toppings (granola, chia seeds, nuts, sliced fruits)

Preparation:

Blend frozen fruits with yogurt and liquid until smooth.

Pour the smoothie into a bowl.

Customize with a variety of toppings for texture and flavor.

Experiment with different fruit combinations and toppings to suit your taste.

Create your signature smoothie bowl that aligns with your cravings and nutritional needs.

These customizable recipes offer a personalized culinary experience, allowing you to take control of your meals and make them uniquely yours. Enjoy the freedom to experiment, adapt, and savor dishes crafted to cater to your individual preferences and dietary requirements.

Chapter 10. Occasional Treats and Indulgences

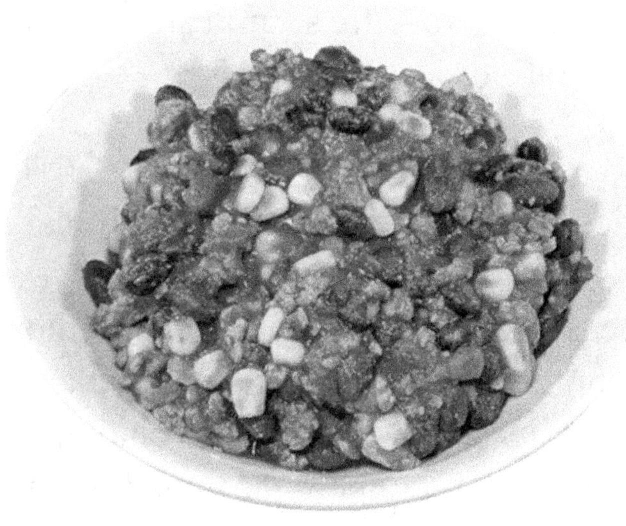

In the final chapter of our culinary journey, we delve into the realm of "Occasional Treats and Indulgences." Here, we embrace the joy that decadent flavors and delightful textures can bring to special moments. While the majority of this cookbook focuses on nourishing and health-conscious recipes, this chapter acknowledges the importance of balance and the occasional indulgence that adds a touch of sweetness to life's milestones and celebrations.

These recipes are crafted with care, inviting you to savor the artistry of occasional treats without compromising on quality or flavor. From luscious desserts to indulgent snacks, each recipe is designed to be a celebration in itself—a moment to be cherished and shared with loved ones.

While the emphasis throughout the book has been on healthful choices, the Occasional Treats chapter recognizes that a well-balanced life includes moments of indulgence. Whether it's a rich chocolate dessert, a decadent cake, or a fancy cocktail, these recipes are meant to be enjoyed mindfully, savoring the experience without guilt.

Indulging in occasional treats isn't just about satisfying cravings; it's about honoring the joyous occasions in our lives. Birthdays, holidays, and milestones deserve to be marked with flavors that linger on the palate and memories that linger in the heart. This chapter provides a collection of recipes that elevate these moments, ensuring that even in indulgence, there is room for mindful enjoyment and appreciation.

So, as you flip through the pages of "Occasional Treats and Indulgences," let it be a reminder that in life's grand tapestry, a dash of indulgence is not only permissible but can be a delightful and integral part of a well-rounded, joy-filled existence.

Conclusion

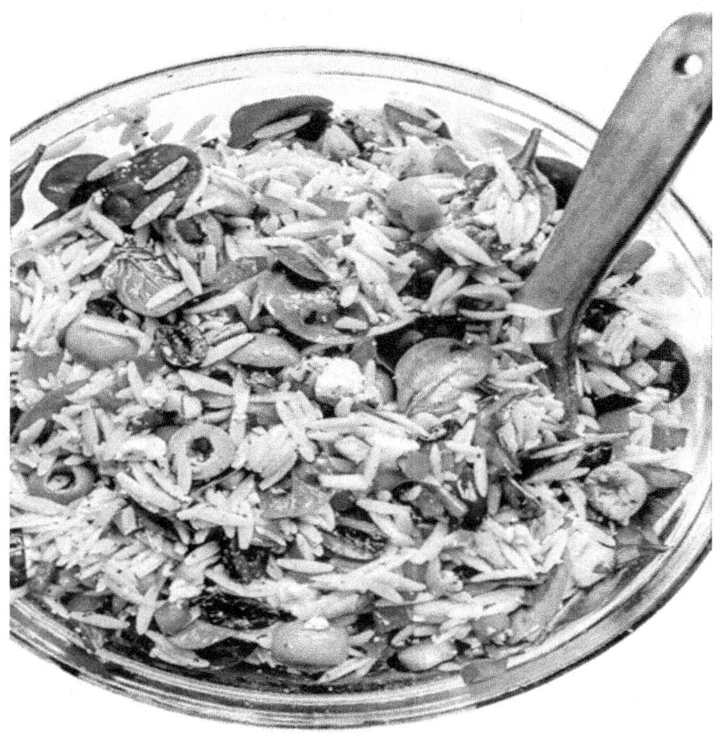

As we draw the curtains on this culinary odyssey, "Beat Cancer Kitchen Cookbook: A Comforting Recipe Guide for Cancer Treatment and Recovery," it's not merely the end of a book but the beginning of a transformative journey.

This cookbook, crafted with passion and purpose, transcends the boundaries of a typical recipe collection. It becomes a companion, a guide, and a source of inspiration for those navigating the challenging terrain of cancer.

Throughout the pages, we've explored the intricate relationship between nutrition and healing, recognizing the profound impact that mindful and purposeful eating can have on the body and soul. From healing broths to nutrient-dense dishes, hydrating elixirs to family-friendly comfort foods, every recipe is a testament to the belief that food is not just sustenance—it is a powerful ally in the fight against cancer.

The heartbeat of this cookbook lies not only in its recipes but in the narrative, it weaves—a narrative of hope, strength, and resilience. It recognizes the significance of family gatherings around a pot of soup, the therapeutic joy of mindful cooking, and the occasional indulgence that adds a touch of sweetness to life's milestones.

In the realm of customizable recipes, we empower individuals to take charge of their nourishment, understanding that every plate is an opportunity for personalization and creativity. The culinary journey presented in this book isn't a rigid set of rules but a flexible and adaptable guide—a source of comfort and empowerment during a time that demands both.

As we bid farewell to the "Beat Cancer Kitchen Cookbook," let it be a reminder that wellness is a holistic pursuit, and every bite can be a step towards healing. May these recipes not only bring nourishment to the body but also comfort to the spirit. Here's to a journey of culinary exploration, a celebration of life, and the hope that, in every kitchen, there is the power to beat cancer one comforting recipe at a time.

Dear Valued Reader,

I hope you enjoyed my book, I poured my heart and soul into it, and I am so grateful that you took the time to read it.

If u found the book helpful, insightful or entertaining, I would be honored If you will consider leaving a positive review. Your feedback means the

world to me as an author, and it can help other potential readers discover my work.

Also, if you think there's are certain contents in the book which you don't really understand, or you have a suggestion towards this book please kindly send me a direct mail here

(larrydanielsbooks@gmail.com)

I will be happy to help and respond